Autoimmune Paleo Cookbook:

Healthy and Easy Anti-Inflammatory Recipes For Healing Autoimmune Disorders and Disease

By

Valerie Alston

Table of Contents

Introduction 5

Carrot Ginger Soup 7

Cream of Broccoli Soup 9

Sweet Potato Salad 12

Fresh Summer Salad 14

Sea Scallops with Mashed Spinach Parsnip 16

Mushroom, Beef, and Ginger Stir-Fry 18

Granola AIP Style 20

Beef Onion Skewers 22

Blueberry Bacon Bars 24

Strawberry Lemon Tart 26

Fermented Sauerkraut Recipe 28

Grilled Lemon Garlic and Rosemary Chicken Breasts 31

Chicken Soup AIP Style 33

Crispy Duck Breast 35

Final Words 37

Thank You Page 38

Autoimmune Paleo Cookbook: Healthy and Easy Anti-Inflammatory Recipes For Healing Autoimmune Disorders and Disease

By Valerie Alston

© Copyright 2014 Valerie Alston

Reproduction or translation of any part of this work beyond that permitted by section 107 or 108 of the 1976 United States Copyright Act without permission of the copyright owner is unlawful. Requests for permission or further information should be addressed to the author.

This publication is designed to provide accurate and authoritative information in regard to the subject matter covered. This work is sold with the understanding that the publisher is not engaged in rendering legal, accounting, or other professional services. If legal advice or other expert assistance is required, the services of a competent professional person should be sought.

First Published, 2014

Printed in the United States of America

Introduction

In today's day and age, many serious changes in health and living have happened over the past few decades and the past century for that matter. Many health programs and diets have been created and practiced over the years to try to battle obesity and for a healthier lifestyle. And speaking of diets, there is one that has become quite a fad at this time and is getting more popular each day, the Paleo Diet and a form of this diet is the Autoimmune Paleo Diet.

The Autoimmune Paleo diet is all about consuming food; it may be fruits, vegetables, and even lean meat that were the same as the food that the Paleolithic humans ate which actually lengthened their life expectancy. Autoimmune diseases stem from a leaky gut that causes different illnesses where the immune system attack the body's cells and therefore make the body weak and prone to other sicknesses and it may be very detrimental to the body and even fatal. These Autoimmune diseases have developed over the years and are now around 80 kinds of autoimmune diseases that plague people all over the world. That is why this

Autoimmune Paleo diet has grown popular because of its promising effects to its practitioners.

There are many various diets to fight these Autoimmune diseases and they are guaranteed to fit your every need from snacks, deserts, main dishes, and even beverages.

Different Recipes for Autoimmune Paleo Diet

Along with the strict compliance to only consuming foods as prescribed by the Paleo Diet, recipes described in this book are some of the most scrumptious, enticingly delicious recipes that will surely get you to try this diet out.

Carrot Ginger Soup

Get a load of a tasty soup to spice up your mornings with the use of some fruits, herbs and even carbohydrates. All these ingredients will definitely make your mouth water and you will crave to have this kind of sour in your table every day.

You can have this soup with wheat bread and as an appetizer for a meal consisting of meat and some fish if you prefer. It can be partnered with chicken as well or lamb. Read up on the instructions below to achieve this mouth-watering soup.

This recipe can serve up to 4 people and can be cooked and prepared in just 1 hour.

What you need:

Peeled and roughly chopped carrots (8)

Peeled and roughly chopped zucchini (2 small pieces)

Minced fresh ginger (2 tablespoons)

Turmeric (1teaspoon)

Diced onion (1 small sized)

Roughly chopped and peeled apple

Cinnamon, just a pinch

Chicken or vegetable stock (4cups)

Cooking oil/fat

Freshly ground black pepper

Rock salt

Coconut milk (1cup/optional)

Steps:

Prepare the cooking fat in the saucepan and wait until melted in medium-high heat.

Sauté the onions and ginger for about 4 minutes. Enjoy the smell of aroma from the pan.

Place all the other ingredients inside the pan and cook until the carrots are soft and cooked. Make sure to stir once in a while to prevent burnt vegetables.

Add the chicken stock and bring to boil in high heat. Let it simmer some more for about 30 minutes.

Using a blender, purée the soup until all are blended and smooth.

Add the coconut oil of you prefer and serve warm to your loved ones.

Cream of Broccoli Soup

This soup will surely warm your cold days and even colder nights. The integration of soups into any type of diet is very beneficial and it will give the necessary additives aside from your main course. This is a version of a cream of broccoli soup which will tickle your taste buds and make you think of a warm cozy bed to snuggle in during winter days.

This recipe serves up to 4 people and takes approximately 55 minutes to cook and prepare.

What you need:

Solid cooking fat (1 tablespoon)

Large yellow onion (1)

Cloves of minced garlic (4)

A large rutabaga which is about ¾ lbs, cut rutabaga into chunks about an inch big

3 cups of bone broth

1 pound broccoli, chopped with florets and stems

Thinly sliced mushrooms (1 cup)

1 cup water

Sea salt (1 teaspoon)

1 garnished avocado

1 can of coconut milk

Steps:

Melt the solid cooking fat in a pan and when the pan is hot, add the chopped onions and cook for about 8 minutes, make sure to stir it until it turns translucent.

Once the onion is translucent in color, add in the garlic and keep stirring for a few more minutes. Make sure not to burn the garlic or it will taste bitter.

Mix in the rutabaga as well as the bone broth and bring to a boil.

Simmer the mixture for about 10 more minutes after boiling. Make sure it is covered and the heat turned low when simmering.

Pour the broccoli, mushrooms, salt and water into the pot and boil again. Once all boiled, turn the heat down again and simmer, cover the pot and cook for another 10-15 minutes or until the vegetables are all soft and tender.

Pour the coconut oil into the pan and mix all ingredients.

Pour in some of the contents, more of the vegetables rather than the soup, into a blender and blend until desired texture.

Put back the blended ingredients into the soup and garnish with fresh avocado. Enjoy!

Sweet Potato Salad

As an appetizer, these sweet potatoes look very promising and yummy which is perfect for every occasion. Potatoes are not allowed in the AIP diet but can be replaced with sweet potatoes instead. You can use maple syrup with this salad as well or better yet, just let the natural sweetness of the sweet potatoes take over. Read up on this recipe for an enjoyable appetizer for the family.

What you need:
2 big sweet potatoes
1 tablespoon bacon fat
¼ cup apple cider vinegar
½ cup green onions, chopped
smoked salt for taste
8 ounces of bacon which is approved by AIP of course

Steps:
Chop the sweet potatoes into small pieces, an inch big is good enough then bake in the oven for about 50 minutes at 35 degrees or until tender using parchment

lined cookie sheets. You can use a spoon to toss it with while it is cooking.

For the bacon, bake it under a 35 degree-heat for about 40 minutes using a cookie sheet as well. Wait until it is brown and crispy.

Mix in vinegar and the bacon fat in a saucepan and cook under medium heat. Cook for about 10 minutes.

Start chopping the bacon into tiny pieces and remove the bottoms of the green onions and mince as well. Set both of them aside and use only ½ cup onions.

Mix the sweet potatoes, chopped bacon, and chopped green onions into a bowl. Remove the bacon and vinegar fat from the heat and pour over the sweet potato mixture. Add salt to taste toss it a bit with a spoon and let the sauce seep in to the ingredients. Serve warm.

Fresh Summer Salad

Eating AIP style can be a bit of a challenge especially with the many limitations and the excluded food from the diet. And the ironic thing is, most of those not allowed to eat are the tastier and delicious ones. It's hard to curb your appetite when you have a variety of food to choose from and it's even harder if you cannot eat them because you are doing AIP.

Fret no more because here's a refreshing salad that will let you forget of those junk food woes and keep you back on track with eating healthy and living longer. So if you want to know more of this garden salad, keep reading.

This salad is very easy to prepare and can serve as many as you want. Just make the necessary adjustments with the measurements. The one shown below specifically just serves 1 person and can be prepared in just 10 minutes.

What you need:

2 sliced whole strawberries

2 cups of mixed greens

½ sliced avocado

¼ cup blueberries

For the dressing:

½ tablespoon of honey

3 tablespoons of extra virgin olive oil

1 tablespoon of Italian Seasoning

1 tablespoon of fresh cilantro

Freshly ground black pepper and sea salt

Steps:

Mix all the ingredients for the dressing in a bowl.

Prepare and mix the salad of berries and cilantro in a plate.

Put the dressing on top and serve.

See, it's as easy as pie so try it now and be on your way to a healthier you!

Sea Scallops with Mashed Spinach Parsnip

It's time for the main course and this dish is one to be remembered because of its great taste and easy preparation. This is perfect for a lovely dinner or brunch which will satisfy all types of hunger and keep you coming back for more.

What you need:

6 diver scallops

2 medium parsnips

2½ cups of baby spinach (organic), washed

2 tablespoons of cultured grass fed organic ghee

Salt

Steps:

Peel off the skins of the parsnips and chop them into pieces, roughly around 2 inches big.

Steam for about 10 minutes or until tender.

Place inside the food processor or blender with the spinach and 1 tablespoon of ghee.

Blend until smooth; don't forget to add salt to taste.

Add 1 tablespoon of ghee into an iron skillet and heat pan until it is hot. Add the scallops into the pan and cook for about 3 minutes.

Prepare a plate of the parsnip and spinach mixture and top it all with the scallops.

Mushroom, Beef, and Ginger Stir-Fry

Are you in the mood for a meaty meal packed with vitamins and nutrients you need for the day? It might be too good to be true for a meaty meal to be nutritious all the way but with the right kind of combinations with vegetables and other natural ingredients, this food heaven can be easily made and achieved in just a few simple steps. If you want to know more about making this and the ingredients needed for this, read on and enjoy.

This recipe serves 4 people and can be prepared and cooked in less than 45 minutes.

What you need:
1 pound of very finely sliced flank steak or sirloin and cut into slim strips
2 minced garlic cloves
Sliced cremini mushrooms (8 oz)
Halved Shitake mushrooms (4oz)
3 cups rapini (broccoli rabe) or chopped kale

Ingredients of Ginger Marinade:

3 tablespoons of rice wine vinegar

1 minced ginger, about the size of a thumb

1 minced garlic clove

¾ cup of beef stock

Freshly ground black pepper and sea salt

Steps:

Mix all the marinade ingredients into a bowl and whisk them all together to combine well.

Place the steak to the marinade and toss gently to mix in further. Put inside the refrigerator for about 15 minutes.

Using a sauté pan, heat some of the cooking fat over a medium- high heat.

Remove just the steak from the marinade mixture. Set aside the marinade mixture. Sauté the steak and garlic in the pan for about 3 to 4 minutes.

Get the steak from the pan and set aside.

Add the kale, mushrooms and the marinade that was set aside and cook for another good 3 to 4 minutes.

Stir in the steak to the mixture after cooking and serve hot.

Granola AIP Style

Want a fancy breakfast with just the right amount of calories but packed with lots of energy? Sounds like the perfect breakfast but it is actually perfect for you. Present the AIP inspired granola for everybody! It's gluten-free and perfect for snacks and just something to nibble on for a quick bite. It will surely keep your stomach feeling full with nutrients. Here's how to make them.

What you need:
2 cups fancy grade coconut flakes
1 tablespoon of coconut oil, heaping
1 tablespoon of coconut manna, heaping
½ teaspoon of cinnamon
Zest of orange
Salt

Steps:
Pour in coconut oil and coconut manna into a pan. Mix in cinnamon after and remove from the heat.
Put coconut flakes in a bowl and spray the coconut oil mix over it. Combine and toss lightly using a spoon.

Zest the orange over the mixture, add a pinch of salt, and stir again carefully.

Lay out evenly the coconut flakes onto a parchment cookie sheet.

Bake the flakes in 350 degrees for about 12-15 minutes. Stir it for a few minutes to avoid turning brown quickly.

Remove from the oven and let it cool. Once cold, serve!

Beef Onion Skewers

This kind of recipe works great with children and is one way of getting them to eat healthy and not be difficult bout it. Try this recipe out and let your kids enjoy this fun and tasty treat.

What you need:
1 pound sirloin steak that are cut into cubes
Coconut aminos (1/4 cup)
1 tablespoon of olive oil
2 tablespoon fresh lemon juice
2 thinly sliced green onions
1 minced glove of garlic
1 tablespoon grated and minced fresh ginger
1 chopped into large pieces red onion
1 tablespoon honey
Freshly ground black pepper and sea salt to taste

Steps:
Mix the olive oil coconut aminos, lemon juice and honey, green onions, salt, garlic, ginger, and pepper to taste in bowl of a marinating container.
Marinate the steak for 2 to 6 hours in the refrigerator.

Preheat grill on a medium-high heat.

Remove the beef from the marinade.

Put the slices of beef and onion slices into the skewers in an alternate manner.

Grill for 10-12 minutes with occasional turning to prevent burnt sides.

Serve immediately.

Blueberry Bacon Bars

Now for a taste of heaven, why not try and make some of this blueberry bacon bars for everybody. This is a fun and exciting way of involving other family members in making this tasty desert.

What you need:
1 ½ cups of sweet potato flour
1 1/3 cup of cultured ghee
¼ cup of coconut oil
1 cup of heaping blueberries
3 pieces of bacon
1 tablespoon of gelatin

Steps:
Cook bacon in a skillet until brown and set aside bacon grease. Allow the bacon to cool and chop it in pieces.
Heat the bacon grease, coconut oil and the cultured ghee in a saucepan.
Whisk and add sweet potato flour into the mixture.
Remove from the heat and add the gelatin and mix the mixture quickly.

Add blueberries and sir again.

Spread this mixture into a dish or bowl and put the chopped bacon on top of the mixture.

Out it inside the refrigerator and let it cool completely.

Take it out of the refrigerator and let it sit for about 10 minutes before serving.

Strawberry Lemon Tart

Another feisty desert to entice the senses and uplift your day, try out this new desert using strawberry and lemon to make the perfect tart. Read up for more information.

What you need:

1 1/3 sweet potato flour

½ cu of coconut oil

1/3 sweet potato flour

½ teaspoon of salt

2 quarts of strawberries

3 tablespoons of maple syrup

3 tablespoons of lemon juice

1 an of cold coconut milk

½ teaspoon of rose water

Steps:

Slice strawberries into pieces which are about 1 inch thick. Put them in a large pot mixing the lemon juice and maple syrup. Cook and bring to simmer for an hour.

Put tapioca and sweet potato flour into the blender; make sure to also add coconut oil and salt and lemon zest. Blend it till the point when mixture is smooth.

In a pan, press the flour into the sides and bottom of the pan and also coat the sides of the pan. Bake the empty tart in the pan for 20 minutes at 350 degrees. Once cooked, take out and let it cool.

Place a strainer over the bowl and carefully pour the hot mixture of the stewed strawberries which took about an hour. Place the strained strawberries in a different bowl.

Place the strawberries into the empty tart and let it cool completely.

Place the top cream of the coconut milk can into a bowl. Add rose water and whip the coconut milk. It can take a few minutes to whip it into a cream.

Slice the tart into separate pieces and garnish with whipped cream!

Fermented Sauerkraut Recipe

What you need:

Lots of Cabbage, about 5 pounds or more if you will store for more people

Sea Salt, 3 tablespoon

Steps:

Wash your equipment thoroughly especially your hands.

Remove the core of the cabbage by cutting it in half. Remove wilted parts as well which are usually the outer layers. Cut the cabbage into quarters and put them all in your food processor. If you don't have a blender or food processor, just cut the cabbage in small pieces. Use the largest blade for the blender for better cutting.

Once it is finely cut and shredded, place it in a large bowl and add the 3 tablespoon sea salt. Toss and mix the salt into the cabbage by using a spoon or ladel.

Transfer the mixed and shredded cabbage into your Fido jar, if there are excess cabbages; just leave them on the plate for later.

Cover the bowl and the jar with cloths and leave them to sweat for about 30 minutes.

After 30 minutes, use a meat pounder or a masher to push down the cabbage into the jar to make room for more cabbages. Mix the remaining cabbages earlier and put the lid back to cover. Let it set for 30 minutes.

After another 30 minutes have passed, push down the cabbage again letting some juices come up on top. If needed, add a little water to make it moist and leave about two inches of space on top of the jar.

Now you are ready to ferment your cabbages. The first week of fermentation is called the gaseous stage. It means that the cabbage will expand upward so if it bubbles, just put a plate on top of the jar. Fido jars are excellent for fermenting because they don't let oxygen inside even if some juices might seep out of the jar. That's fine, it is better than oxygen getting into the jar. That will cause molds to build and ruin your fermented cabbage

Label the jar with the date that you made it and let it ferment for 30 days. Put it in a cold dry place and take care not to expose it to sunlight or to oxygen. The fermentation duration also depends on the temperature of your house. If it is during the summer and the inside of your house is hot, ferment the cabbage for only 3 weeks. If it is during cold seasons, ferment it in 5 weeks.

The best temperatures for fermentation is between 60-75 degrees so don't let it go beyond 80 degrees or it will just go bad.

Once required time has passed, place the cabbage in smaller bottles and put in the fridge for consumption. They should be good for 6 months if refrigerated.

Grilled Lemon Garlic and Rosemary Chicken Breasts

What you need:

Boneless chicken breasts, 2 pounds

Half cup of freshly squeezed lemon juice

1 tablespoon extra virgin olive oil

1 pressed garlic clove

1 tablespoon fresh rosemary, minced

¼ teaspoon sea salt

¼ teaspoon black pepper

Steps:

Get a large glass measuring cup, mix the ingredients of olive oil, rosemary, lemon juice, garlic, salt and pepper. Leave and set aside for later.

Pound the chicken until even and then cut it into strips. Place the chicken on a flat dish and pour the marinade in top. Cover well and coat all parts. Refrigerate for 2 to 3 hours. Do not go over 3 hours because the lemon juice is strong and might ruin the taste if left on for longer.

Gas grill must be preheated for about 10 minutes. Turn the heat down to medium and grill the chicken strips, cover and cook for 4 minutes on each side.

Chicken Soup AIP Style

What you need:

1 whole chicken it has to be organic and about 3 to 4 pounds

2-3 large onions, they have to be peeled and quartered

6 stalks of rinsed and halved celery

6 scrubbed and halved carrots

6 peeled cloves of garlic

4 pieces of ginger, peeled and quarter

1 tablespoons apple cider vinegar

4 tablespoons of unrefined coconut oil

2 tablespoons of sea salt

4-6 cups of water

4 cups of thinly sliced carrots

1 pound of frozen peas

Steps:

Place all the ingredients in a large soup pot except the water, thinly sliced carrots and the peas. Fill it with water and bring to boil. Once it reached its boiling point, turn down heat and simmer for 8 hours. Add water as you simmer it for 8 hours so it won't dry out.

Use two large spoons to lift the chicken and set aside in a plate. Do not use a thong because the chicken might fall apart.

Strain the stock in a different bowl and pour the stock back into the soup pot. Throw away the vegetables that were boiled, they no longer have any nutritional value.

Gather the meat from the chicken and throw away the bones because they no longer have any nutrients in them.

Add more water to the pot, about 4-6 cups, add the thinly sliced carrots and bring to a simmer.

When the carrots are a bit tender, add the peas and simmer for another 2 minutes. For strict API compliance, you can substitute the peas with broccoli.

Crispy Duck Breast

Here's a treat for those who don't want to sacrifice their meat and still be on the healthy side. This serves two persons but you can adjust the servings by adding to the ingredient amount.

What you need:
2 duck breasts
Sea salt

Steps:
With a paper towel, pat the duck breast dry gently. Make sure the paper towel does not leave any paper on the duck breasts.
With a sharp knife, cut the skin in crosshatches or in a pattern. Make sure the skin is penetrated but not too deep that it cuts through the skin. The crosshatch pattern will ensure the fat between the skin and the meet will be cooked.
Sprinkle both sides of the duck breasts with an ample amount of sea salt Place them into a skillet with the skin facing downwards. The skillet must be cold and dry and leave it uncovered.

Turn the heat into medium and set your timer into 15 minutes. Keep an eye on it because the skin might be burned if heat is too high. This amount of time is an approximate time for the fat to be burned and for the skin to turn nice and crispy.

Once the skin looks crispy enough, turn it to the other side and cook for another 5 minutes.

Once cooked, remove from the pan and set for 5 minutes. Cut the duck meat into diagonal slices.

Add any vegetable to this dish and serve hot.

Final Words

So there you go! These are just some of the many recipes of the Autoimmune Paleo Diet which you can have from breakfast, to lunch and all the way to dinner and desert. Even if you are on a certain type of diet, doesn't mean you should starve yourself. You just need to regulate your food intake and totally avoid some foods that are not AIP friendly.

These are the things you need to know about the Autoimmune Paleo Diet and why people are getting into this type of weight-loss program. It is not actually primarily about weight loss, it is about eating the right kind of food which was patterned from our ancestors' time during the Paleolithic era.

If you are plagued by ailments of the digestive system and the leaky gut, make sure to read up on this alternative diet and learn how it can benefit you and your health over time.

Thank You Page

I want to personally thank you for reading my book. I hope you found information in this book useful and I would be very grateful if you could leave your honest review about this book. I certainly want to thank you in advance for doing this.

CPSIA information can be obtained
at www.ICGtesting.com
Printed in the USA
LVOW04s0026071216
516143LV00028BA/594/P